Fundoscopy Made Easy

Sujoy Ghosh MD DM MRCP(UK) MRCPS(Glas),
Clinical Teaching and Clinical Research Fellow,
The Ayr Hospital, Ayr, UK

Andrew Collier BSc(Hons) MBChB MD FRCP(Edin&Glas),
Honorary Senior Lecturer and Consultant Physician,
The Ayr Hospital, Ayr, UK

Mohan Varikkara MS FRCS(Edin),
Consultant Ophthalmologist, The Ayr Hospital, Ayr, UK

Stephen Palmer MIMI RMIP,
Head of Department, Medical Photography
and Audiovisual Services, NHS Ayrshire & Arran, UK

Foreword by
Neil Dewhurst MD FRCPE FRCP FRCPG
President, Royal College of Physicians, Edinburgh, UK

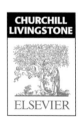

CHURCHILL
LIVINGSTONE

ELSEVIER

D1334310

Edinburgh   London   New York   Oxford   Philadelphia   St Louis   Sydney   Toronto 2010

CHURCHILL
LIVINGSTONE
ELSEVIER

ISBN 978-0-7020-4297-3
International ISBN 978-0-7020-4298-0

British Library Cataloguing in Publication Data
A catalogue record for this book is available from the British Library.

Library of Congress Cataloging in Publication Data
A catalog record for this book is available from the Library of Congress.

Notices
Knowledge and best practice in this field are constantly changing. As new research and experience broaden our understanding, changes in research methods, professional practices, or medical treatment may become necessary.

Practitioners and researchers must always rely on their own experience and knowledge in evaluating and using any information, methods, compounds, or experiments described herein. In using such information or methods they should be mindful of their own safety and the safety of others, including parties for whom they have a professional responsibility.

With respect to any drug or pharmaceutical products identified, readers are advised to check the most current information provided (i) on procedures featured or (ii) by the manufacturer of each product to be administered, to verify the recommended dose or formula, the method and duration of administration, and contraindications. It is the responsibility of practitioners, relying on their own experience and knowledge of their patients, to make diagnoses, to determine dosages and the best treatment for each individual patient, and to take all appropriate safety precautions.

To the fullest extent of the law, neither the Publisher nor the authors, contributors, or editors, assume any liability for any injury and/or damage to persons or property as a matter of products liability, negligence or otherwise, or from any use or operation of any methods, products, instructions, or ideas contained in the material herein.

Printed in China

CONTENTS

FOREWORD

It is a pleasure to be invited to contribute a foreword for 'Fundoscopy Made Easy'. Acquiring knowledge and mastering clinical skills remain core to training at both undergraduate and postgraduate level. Perfecting and maintaining the skills involved in ophthalmoscopy remain challenging for most doctors in training. In this respect the introductory chapters on equipment, techniques and normal findings take the reader in an orderly fashion through the basics. Over the years technology has advanced and the descriptions of the newer techniques for visualising the retina are important even for the nonspecialist.

The sequence of the following chapters takes the reader through a systematic and comprehensive review of the various retinal pathologies. The layout is consistent between chapters and makes the whole text highly readable with an appropriate level of detail related to not only diagnosis but also treatment options for the various conditions. I am sure all readers will be impressed by the quality of the image reproduction. The authors are to be congratulated on producing a volume which is more than simply an atlas of pathology.

At a time when we all run the risk of becoming de-skilled in fundal examination, this book's publication is timely. It will be particularly useful for all trainees in both primary and secondary care, especially for those who may be studying for College examinations. It is a highly readable text and I hope you enjoy it as much as I have.

Neil Dewhurst

PREFACE

Examination of the fundus is an area where the non-specialist often has limited knowledge. Medical students, junior doctors and physicians (whatever grade) need to have a basic knowledge of fundal examination, irrespective of the speciality that they are working in. In today's changing educational curriculum there is less opportunity for all concerned to master this art. Although there are several textbooks on ophthalmology and fundoscopy, very few are targeted at the needs of medical students and junior doctors.

This book has been specifically designed to fill that gap and make fundoscopy and interpretation of fundal images as simple as possible. Often making a diagnosis on fundoscopy is like 'matching wallpaper'. Once you have seen one you can identify it when you see it again. The high-quality images provided in this book, together with concise write-ups, should provide the core knowledge required not only for medical students and junior doctors but also for doctors in training preparing for examinations (including the MRCP). It will also be useful for optometrists and medical photographers.

This book in not meant to be an alternative to conventional textbooks or the expert opinion of an ophthalmologist, but should be able to provide the reader with enough information to help identify/diagnose the most common retinal abnormalities.

S. Ghosh
A. Collier
M. Varikarra
S. Palmer

ACKNOWLEDGMENTS

For valuable assistance preparing and sourcing the many Illustrations, the authors would like to thank Sarah Syme, Valerie Wyllie, David Dickie, Wendy Trainor and Emma Lehane from NHS Ayrshire & Arran's Medical Photography department, John McCormick, Iain Smith and Prof Gordon Dutton, from the Tennent Institute of Ophthalmology at Gartnavel General Hospital, Glasgow, and Colin Clements from Kings College Hospital, London.

We would like to thank Margaret McMurdo for her help preparing the manuscript.

DIGITAL RETINAL PHOTOGRAPHY AND THE IMAGES IN THIS BOOK

Most, if not all, of the photographs in this book were taken with Topcon digital retinal cameras. Within the authors' workplace these are predominantly the Topcon TRC-NW6 fitted with a Nikon D70 camera back. This is a non-mydriatic camera which does not usually require the patient's eyes to be dilated; however, a much greater success rate can be achieved if tropicamide or similar mydriatic eye drops are used. Non-mydriatic cameras operate by using an infrared-sensitive video camera image to position and focus the image of the retina. As no visible light is used, the patient's pupil will not constrict, and a photograph can then be taken using the built-in flash. The flash duration is so short that the exposure is made before the pupil can react.

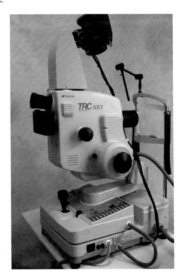

Mydriatic photographs taken within the Ophthalmology Department were produced using either a Topcon TRC-50EX or a Canon CF-60 mydriatic camera. In this way, a 45-degree area of the retina can be covered by each photograph. The Topcon TRC-NW6 incorporates one central and eight fixed peripheral internal fixation points. Using each of these fixation points will cover 85 degrees of the retina. The cen-

Topcon Fundus Camera

tral fixation point allows a repeatable photograph of the posterior pole. This is the basic image used for the Scottish Diabetic Retinal Screening Programme.

CHAPTER 1

The Basics: Direct and Indirect Ophthalmoscopy

The direct ophthalmoscope is the instrument of choice for fundus examination by medical students and physicians. It allows for a magnified, monocular image of the retina and optic disc.

Principle

The instrument illuminates the subject's fundus by light reflected off a mirror on the instrument head. A perforation in the centre of the mirror helps the observer view the area illuminated. The emanating rays from the subject's eyes are parallel, assuming the subject is emmetropic (normal sighted). These rays are converged to a focus (assuming the observer is also normal sighted) by the observer's cornea and crystalline lens onto the observer's retina. The emanating rays from a myopic subject's eye would be convergent and therefore will require a concave lens to make it parallel before entering

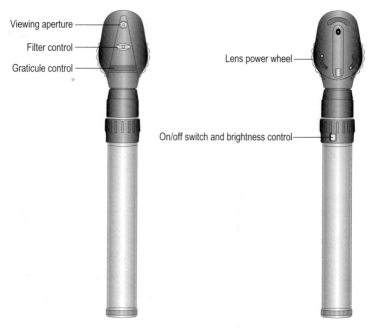

The ophthalmoscope.

the observer's eye and the converse if the subject is hyperopic. These lenses are mounted on a wheel on the ophthalmoscope head which can be dialled appropriately.

Methods

If you are using an unfamiliar ophthalmoscope it would help to familiarise yourself with the colour coding of the lens wheel and the various apertures and filters. To undertake successful ophthalmoscopy it is essential that both you and the patient are comfortable. Adjust the height of the patient in such a way that you don't have to stoop too much. Dim the main lights to allow for physiological mydriasis if the pupil is not pharmacologically dilated. Tropicamide 1% is a short-acting dilator which can be used safely unless contraindicated by allergy or due to a shallow anterior chamber which may precipitate an acute glaucoma on dilation of the pupil. A shallow chamber can be reasonably assessed by using a pen light that is shone from the side of the cornea, parallel to the iris. Normally the opposite half of the iris beyond the pupil should be illuminated by your light. If it is shadowed, the configuration of the iris is considered convex, thus indicating a shallow anterior chamber.

Instruct the patient to look at a distant target. Let the patient know that they can blink if required. Stand at the side of the patient. Ideally use your left eye and left hand to examine the patient's left eye. Rest your free hand on the patient's forehead, using your thumb to hold the upper lid open if necessary. Use only the minimum required intensity of light. The field of view of the fundus is increased the closer you are to the patient's eye. For low myopes and low hyperopes it is best to remove their spectacles; however, for high myopes, hyperopes and for subjects with high astigmatism it is advisable to keep the spectacles on in order to overcome problems associated with magnification, minification or distortion, respectively. The extra reflexes produced by the spectacle lenses may at first prove distracting but can be overcome with practice.

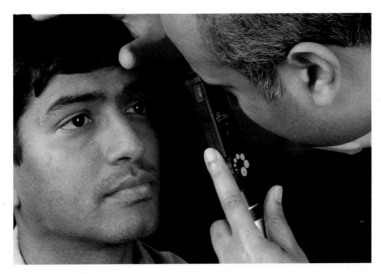

Examination by direct ophthalmoscope.

Examination of the red reflex

Start the examination by doing a 'distant direct' ophthalmoscopy from a distance of 30 cm using a plano lens in the aperture of the ophthalmoscope. This technique is used to study the red reflex and each eye should be compared. While examining the red reflex, ask the patient to look up or down slightly. If, when the patient looks up, the opacity appears to move in the same direction within the red reflex, then it must lie anterior to the pupil plane (i.e. the cornea or the anterior chamber). One that remains stationary must be in the plane of the pupil and one that moves in the opposite direction to that of the patient's gaze must lie posterior to the pupil plane (i.e. the posterior lens or vitreous). You may find it easier to move yourself slightly up or down rather than ask the patient to move their eye to achieve the same effect.

During ophthalmoscopy it is advisable to keep both eyes open and suppress the image from the other eye. This reduces the effect of accommodation. It may take some practice to accomplish this.

Examination of the optic disc

Slowly move closer to the patient and at the same time gradually increase the power of the lens in the wheel to focus on the retina. The power necessary to focus on the fundus will depend on both the patient's and the observer's uncompensated refractive error and their accommodation. When the patient is looking straight ahead, the optic disc should naturally come into the field of view. If not, try to locate a blood vessel on the retina and then move along it and locate the point at which it branches. Move your field of view in the direction in which the apex of the branch is pointing. By moving along a blood vessel in this manner the optic disc will be located. You will need to consider its colour, clear definition of its margins, cup (if there is one) and the ratio of the size of the cup to the size of the optic disc (cup disc ratio, denoted as, e.g., 0.3:1, meaning it occupies one-third of the area of the optic disc). Note the capillaries on the optic disc and look for the presence of a spontaneous venous pulsation. Also note the presence of any pigment, choroidal or scleral crescents around the disc.

Examination of the retinal blood vessels

Retinal blood vessels should be examined by following the temporal and nasal arcades from the optic disc. Veins are larger and dark red, whereas arteries are relatively thinner and lighter (normal artery:vein ratio is 2:3).

Examination of the macula

The macula is visualised by asking the patient to look at the light source as this brings the fovea (fixation point) into view. The macula is the area between the superior and inferior temporal arcades and its centre is the fovea. Since using an excessively bright light can make the macula difficult to visualise, it may be useful to use a smaller aperture beam and minimal required intensity.

Examination of the peripheral fundus

Finally, ask the patient to look in the eight cardinal directions to allow you to view the peripheral fundus – 'Look up', to see the superior periphery and so on. You will need to adjust the lens in the wheel slightly as the periphery is closer to you than the optic disc, requiring more focusing power.

Indirect ophthalmoscopy

Binocular indirect ophthalmoscopy

This technique allows for viewing the fundus at a wider angle which allows examination of the peripheral retina and also a better view through lens opacities as well. Binocularity is achieved by the use of mirrors in the instrument to reduce the pupillary distance of the observer to about 15 mm. The instrument also carries a light source which is attached to a headband or spectacle frame worn by the examiner.

The patient's pupil may be dilated and background lights dimmed as for direct ophthalmoscopy. The patient is examined either seated in a reclining chair or lying on a couch. A condensing lens (varying from +15 D to +30 D) is held in one hand of the examiner in front of the patient's eye. The image formed is magnified three-fold with a 20 D lens and is inverted and laterally reversed (superior seen inferiorly and temporal seen nasally).

Ensure that the patient's and the observer's eye are aligned before placing the lens in front of the eye. Check for the red reflex first and then bring the condensing lens in front of the patient's eye. Now

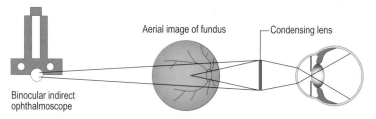

The binocular indirect ophthalmoscope.

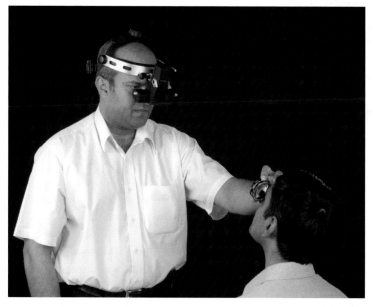

Examination by indirect ophthalmoscope.

gradually pull the lens towards you until the whole lens is filled with the retinal image. Systematically view the patient's fundus in primary and all secondary positions of gaze. Also remember to compare the two eyes. The ora serrata can be viewed by scleral indentation with the free hand of the observer under local anaesthetic (proxymetacaine). It is important to remember that you are viewing the superior retina when the patient is looking up despite the image being inverted and laterally reversed, and this relationship is maintained for the other quadrants.

Slit lamp biomicroscopy

The fundus also can be viewed by using a non-contact Volk condensing lens (+60 to +90 D) or a Goldmann contact lens (–64 D) and the slit lamp. This is the most common method of examination of the fundus dilated or undilated at the ophthalmology clinic. The patient's pupil may be dilated and background lights dimmed as for direct ophthalmoscopy.

Once the patient is positioned comfortably at the slit lamp, the patient is advised to look straight ahead and not into the light (ask the patient to look at the examiner's right ear with the left eye while examining the patient's right eye and vice versa). The slit lamp viewing piece and the light column are kept at an angle of 90 degrees. The intensity of the beam is kept to the minimum possible and the magnification preferably set at 10× initially. The slit beam is set around 1.5–2.5 mm wide and 5–10 mm long. The beam is focused onto the patient's pupil and the condensing lens aligned at around 1 cm from the patient's eye. The slit lamp is then pulled backwards gradually towards the examiner until it comes into focus with the aerial image of the fundus between the condensing lens and the slit lamp. Alternatively, the slit lamp could be drawn back completely towards the examiner and then gradually moved forwards until the image comes into focus.

As with indirect ophthalmoscopy, the image from a non-contact Volk lens slit lamp biomicroscopic examination is inverted and laterally reversed. The fundus is viewed systematically in primary and all secondary positions of gaze. The ora serrata can be brought to view using the Goldmann three-mirror lens.

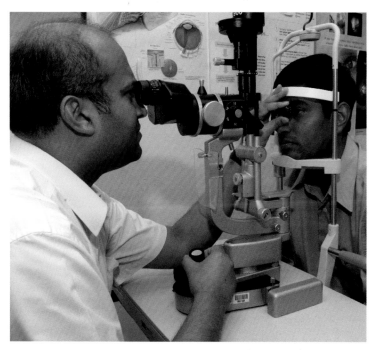

Examination by slit lamp biomicroscopy.

CHAPTER 2

Specialised Imaging Techniques

In addition to binocular indirect ophthalmoscopy and slit lamp biomicroscopy described in Chapter 1, the following specialised imaging techniques are useful in diagnosing particular conditions.

Fundal fluorescein angiography (FFA)

Fluorescein angiography is a technique often used for examining the circulation of the retina. It involves injection of sodium fluorescein dye into the systemic circulation. A series of images are then obtained by photographing the fluorescence emitted after illumination of the retina with blue light.

Some staining of the skin is visible about 5 minutes after dye injection. The fluorescein dye is cleared by the kidney in 12–24 hours. Some patients experience nausea which is typically transient. Allergic reactions are uncommon. The reaction can range from a minor annoyance to a severe reaction. Anaphylactic shock following an injection of sodium fluorescein dye is very rare. However, it is important to ensure that a suitably equipped emergency trolley is available.

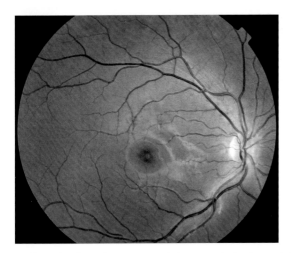

Red free: Blood vessels are seen as dark against the background of normal fundus reflectance with striations from the retinal nerve fibre layer.

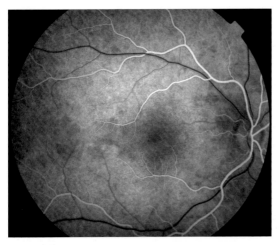

11.1 sec: Choroidal filling which is the earliest, is seen as the grey background. The dye has now filled the retinal arteries and is starting to show laminar flow in the retinal veins.

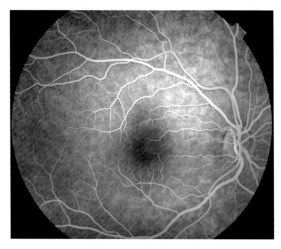

133 sec: The next phase shows emptying of retinal arteries and full retinal veins. Note the fine perifoveal capillary network.

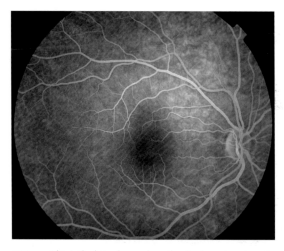

342 sec: This is the late phase where the dye has already recirculated. Note the staining of the optic nerve head and extravasated dye in the choroidal spaces.

Technique

- Baseline colour and monochrome red-free (green filter) images are taken prior to injection. This allows for the visualisation of autofluorescence of the retinal tissues.
- A bolus of approximately 5 cc of 10% sodium fluorescein is injected into a suitable vein in the arm or the back of the hand.
- A blue filter is placed before the photography light source. This has the effect of exciting the fluorescein dye, which in turn produces yellow–green (530 nm) light.
- A barrier filter is placed in front of the camera. This ensures that only the yellow–green fluorescence is recorded.
- The fluorescein dye reaches the retinal circulation approximately 10 seconds after injection. A series of black and white digital photographs are taken of the retina to capture the different phases of the dye in the choroidal and retinal circulation. Late images are obtained at 5 and 10 minutes.
- Black and white photographs give a better contrast than colour photographs, as only light of a very narrow wavelength is being transmitted though the barrier filter.

Indocyanine green (ICG) angiography

Indocyanine green is the second dye used in angiography. It fluoresces less than fluorescein sodium and does so at 835 nm. It is also a relatively larger molecule and is 98% bound to plasma proteins. As such, it does not leak as easily as fluorescein sodium from the choroidal vessels and therefore delineates them well. It is not metabolized and is filtered out by the liver and excreted in the bile.

The images that follow illustrate the mid phase of an ICG angiogram and show well-delineated choroidal vasculature of both eyes.

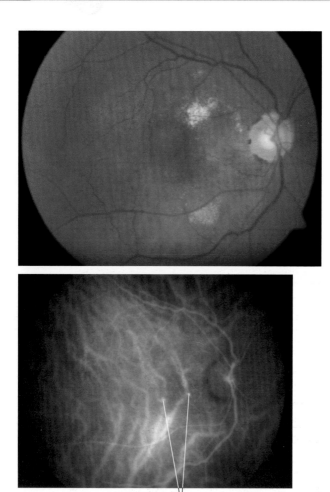

Hyperfluorescent spots

ICG angiogram. Note the two hyperfluorescent spots (arrowed) responsible for the exudative changes seen in the colour image above.

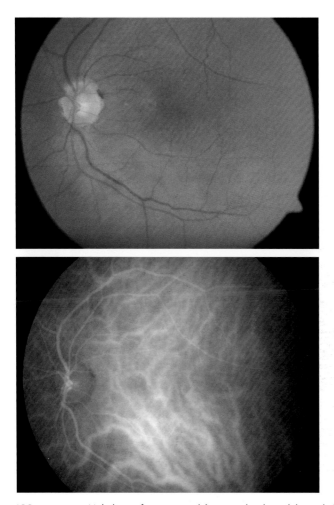

ICG angiogram. Mid phase of angiogram delineating the choroidal vessels (colour picture of the same eye seen above).

Optical coherence tomography (OCT)

Optical coherence tomography is a medical diagnostic imaging technology that provides detailed cross-sectional or tomographic imaging of biological tissues. Unlike ultrasound scans, this device relies on light rather than sound waves. It permits simultaneous viewing of the position on the ocular structure as well as its high-resolution transverse cross-section/three-dimensional image. It allows for both anterior and posterior segment high-resolution imaging.

The OCT signal from a particular tissue layer is a combination of its reflectivity and absorption characteristics combined with the scattering properties of its overlying layers. The nerve fibre layer forms the inner boundary and the retinal pigment epithelium forms the outer boundary of the retina. High reflective layers are represented by red and white colours while lower reflective layers are represented by blue and black colours. OCT therefore helps in diagnosing minimal disturbances in structural integrity. Its ability to quantify change combined with excellent reproducibility makes it an invaluable tool to monitor changes.

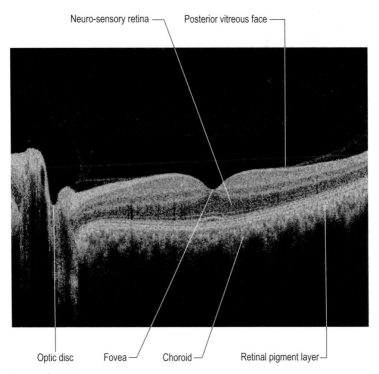

Neuro-sensory retina —   Posterior vitreous face —

Optic disc   Fovea —   Choroid —   Retinal pigment layer —

A normal OCT image.

CHAPTER 3

The Normal Fundus and Its Variants

Macula

Anatomically the macula is the area centred within the temporal arcades measuring about 5.5 mm (3.5 disc diameter, DD).

Fovea

The fovea is a concavity in the centre of the macula measuring about 1.5 mm or 1.0 DD. It is the most sensitive part of the retina, serving the function of high spatial resolution and colour vision. On fundoscopy, due to its concavity, a fovea maintaining its normal architecture shows a bright reflex known as the foveal reflex.

Foveola

A central 0.35 mm of the fovea is known as the foveal avascular zone (FAZ) of the retina as it is free of retinal capillaries. This area consists purely of cone photoreceptors and no overlying inner layers of the retina.

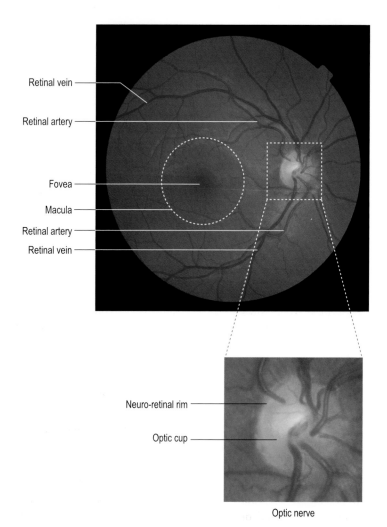

Retinal vein

Retinal artery

Fovea

Macula

Retinal artery

Retinal vein

Neuro-retinal rim

Optic cup

Optic nerve

A normal fundus.

Retinal arteries

The walls of the retinal blood vessels are transparent and therefore we see the column of blood flowing in them. On fundoscopy, the arteries appear lighter and narrower (arteriovenous ratio of 2:3) compared to the retinal veins. The central retinal artery emerges at the optic disc and divides into four branches (superotemporal, inferotemporal, superonasal and inferonasal). In the retina they divide dichotomously until third-order branches finally form a two-tier perivenular capillary network. The superior branches respect the horizontal raphe and normally do not communicate with the inferior branches. The retinal capillary wall is lined by endothelial cells and pericytes which form a tight inner retinal barrier. The retinal blood vessels are autoregulated like those of the brain.

Retinal veins

The perivenular capillaries ultimately form the four main branches (superotemporal, inferotemporal, superonasal and inferonasal) before forming the central retinal vein at the optic disc. The vessels cross over one another in the retina.

The optic disc

Measuring about 1.5 mm, the optic disc lies about 3 mm nasal to the fovea. The edge of the optic disc may be slightly elevated. The immediate peripapillary area may show hyperpigmentation or a scalloped pale area representing the sclera, seen through the transparent retina. The only neuroretinal elements at the optic disc are the axons of the ganglion cells which make up the neuroretinal rim. The central part, the optic cup, occupying around 30% of the entire optic disc area, is paler and appears depressed on binocular stereo fundoscopy. The central retinal vessels enter and leave in this depression. Spontaneous venous pulsations are often seen at the optic disc; however, they may be absent in around 20% of normal individuals. The optic disc also has small capillaries. Physiologically the optic disc represents the blind spot.

Normal fundus variants

Tigroid

In a tigroid fundus there are lesser amounts of pigment in the retinal pigment epithelium, allowing streaks of underlying normal choroidal pigmentation to become visible and give the characteristic appearance.

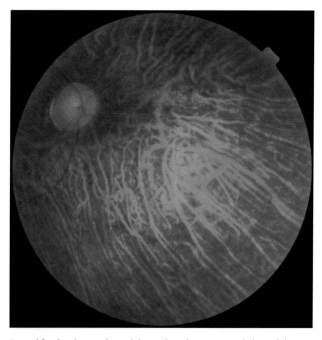

Tigroid fundus: larger choroidal vessels with interspersed choroidal pigment showing through.

Myelinated nerve fibres

Myelinated nerve fibres are relatively common and may follow several patterns:

- Isolated peripheral patch of myelination.
- Pericapillary myelination may be mistaken for papilloedema on examination.
- The myelinated nerve fibres follow the pattern of normal fibres and extend as regular, feather-like patches, which may or may not obscure the retinal blood vessel. Although myelination usually remains stationary, it may very well disappear in optic atrophy following either optic neuritis or ischaemia. It may be associated with neurofibromatosis-1.

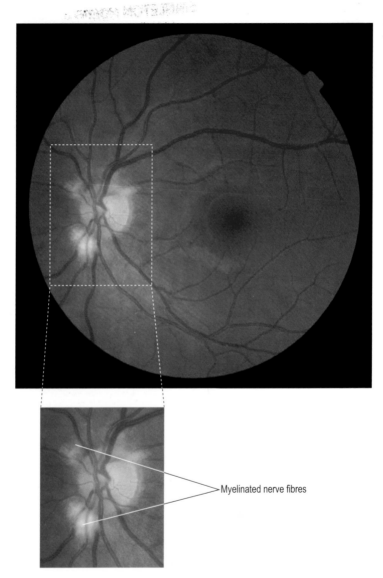

Myelinated nerve fibres

Myelinated nerve fibres. Note the pale appearance adjacent to the optic disc corresponding to arrangement or pattern of retinal nerve fibres.

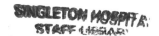

Albino fundus

Melanocytes normally synthesise melanin in the retinal pigment epithelium. Absence of melanin due to any defect in its synthesis allows the choroidal vasculature to be seen under the retinal vessels.

Ocular albinism is a rare X-linked disorder, affecting the eyes only.

Oculocutaneous albinism is an autosomal recessive condition, characterised by hypopigmentation of skin, hair, fundus and irides. It is often associated with a decrease in visual acuity, photophobia and nystagmus.

Such patients may be classified as tyrosinase positive or negative, with the degree of pigmentation usually being greater in tyrosinase-positive patients.

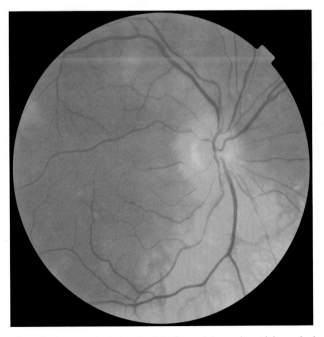

Albino fundus: note the lighter fundal reflex with large choroidal vessels showing through. Absence of normal macular pigmentation and loss of foveal reflex represents macular hypoplasia.

Artefacts in the normal fundus

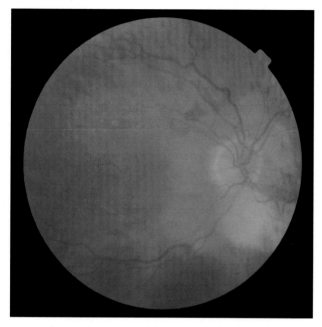

Note eye lash artefact inferior to the optic disc.

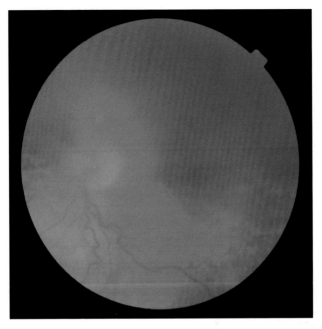

Blurred fundus image due to media opacity caused by cataract.

CHAPTER 4

Diabetic Retinopathy

Diabetic retinopathy is more likely to occur in patients who have poorly controlled diabetes and its prevalence increases with the duration of the diabetes. In type 1 diabetic patients, 50% will have some form of retinopathy after 10 years. Approximately 5–10% of type 2 diabetic patients will have retinopathy at the time of diagnosis of diabetes. Other risk factors for diabetic retinopathy include hypertension, renal disease, obesity, dyslipidaemia, pregnancy, smoking and anaemia. Microvascular leakage and non-perfusion are the main aetiopathogenic processes. The tight junction of the endothelial cells constitutes the inner blood–retinal barrier. Pericytes wrapped round the capillaries are thought to be responsible for the structural integrity of the blood vessels. In diabetic patients there is a reduction in pericytes and endothelial cells, leading to a breakdown of this barrier.

Classification of diabetic retinopathy

Conventionally, involvement of the retina in patients with diabetes has been classified as non-proliferative (background) retinopathy, pre-proliferative retinopathy and proliferative retinopathy. The macula may be involved (maculopathy) with any of the above forms of retinopathy.

A commonly used grading system is that of the Early Treatment Diabetic Retinopathy Study (ETDRS) (Table 4.1).

Table 4.1 Early treatment diabetic retinopathy study system

Grade	Features
Non-proliferative diabetic retinopathy (NPDR)	
None	Normal retina
Early	Microaneurysms only
Mild	Microaneurysms plus: • Retinal haemorrhages, and/or • Hard exudates (> 2 DD from fovea)
Moderate	Mild; NPDR plus: • Haemorrhage and/or cotton wool spots (< 5), and/or • Minimal venous beading/looping or IRMAs in one quadrant
Severe 4/2/1 rule	Moderate; NPDR plus • Microaneurysms/haemorrhages in four quadrants, or • Venous beading/looping in two or more quadrants, or • IRMAs in one quadrant
Very severe	Any two or more of the 'severe categories'
Proliferative diabetic retinopathy (PDR)	
PDR without high-risk changes	NVE or NVD <½ DD
PDR with high-risk changes	NVE or NVD >½ DD plus pre-retinal and/or vitreous haemorrhages

IRMAs, intraretinal microvascular abnormalities; NVD, neovascularisation of the disc; NVE, neovascularisation elsewhere.

Table 4.1 Early treatment diabetic retinopathy study system—Cont'd

Disease severity level	Findings observable on dilated ophthalmoscopy
Diabetic macular oedema apparently absent	No apparent retinal thickening or hard exudates in posterior pole
Diabetic macular oedema apparently present	Some apparent retinal thickening or hard exudates in posterior pole
Mild diabetic macular oedema	Some retinal thickening or hard exudates in posterior pole but distant from the centre of the macula
Moderate diabetic macular oedema	Retinal thickening or hard exudates approaching the centre of the macula but not involving the centre
Severe diabetic macular oedema	Retinal thickening or hard exudates involving the centre of the macula

Non-proliferative (background) diabetic retinopathy

Microaneurysms are the first clinically detectable lesions and represent a dilated part of the perivenular capillaries. They occur due to a reduction in the number of endothelial cells and pericytes, appearing as tiny round dots anywhere in the retina. Intraretinal haemorrhages can be dot or blot if they lie in the deeper compact layers of the retina, or flame shaped if they lie in the nerve fibre layer (obeying the arrangement of the nerve fibres). Hard exudates appear yellow and waxy with relatively distinct margins and represent intraretinal deposition of serum lipids. They usually border the normal and oedematous retina, are usually found in the posterior pole and can often be seen in a circinate pattern around a cluster of microaneurysms. Retinal oedema represents leaky capillaries and is often difficult to delineate with direct ophthalmoscopy. It should always be suspected in the presence of hard exudates. Visual acuity declines if the retinal oedema involves the fovea.

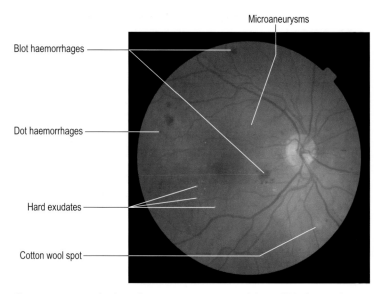

Microaneurysms

Blot haemorrhages

Dot haemorrhages

Hard exudates

Cotton wool spot

There are numerous hard exudates, microaneurysms and dot and blot haemorrhages which are characteristic of background diabetic retinopathy.

Pre-proliferative diabetic retinopathy

Pre-proliferative diabetic retinopathy develops in eyes that initially may only show simple background retinopathy; it is caused by retinal ischaemia. Pre-proliferative diabetic retinopathy is characterised by:

- *Vascular changes* consisting of venous changes in the form of 'beading', 'looping' and 'sausage-like' segmentation. The arterioles may also be narrowed and even obliterated, resembling a branch retinal artery occlusion.
- *Cotton wool spots* caused by interruption of axoplasmic flow caused by the ischaemia, and subsequent build-up of transported material within the nerve axons, is responsible for the white appearance of these lesions.

- *Dark blot haemorrhages* represent haemorrhagic retinal infarcts.
- *Intraretinal microvascular abnormalities (IRMAs)* represent either dilated pre-existing vessels or early intraretinal new vessels. They are found within an area of capillary non-perfusion.

As pre-proliferative changes suggest increasing retinal ischaemia and precede proliferative retinopathy, the patient should be informed of the worsening of their retinopathy and the likely need for laser photocoagulation in the future. The presence of ischaemic maculopathy should be assessed as it could lead to irreversible loss of vision.

A grading system for screening for diabetic retinopathy, and guidelines for specialist assessment, are outlined in Tables 4.2 and 4.3, respectively.

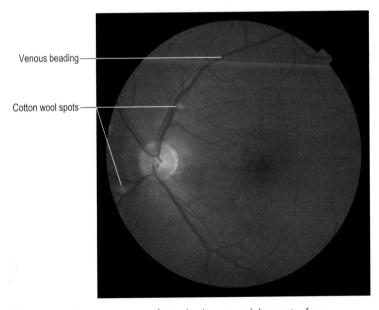

The abnormalities are suggestive of retinal ischaemia and diagnostic of pre-proliferative diabetic retinopathy, the forerunner of neovascularisation. These patients should be referred for specialist assessment and close follow-up.

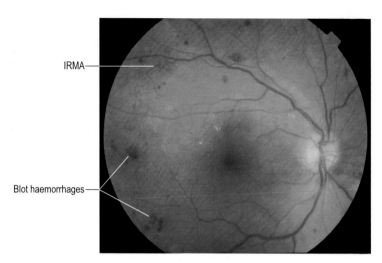

Pre-proliferative diabetic retinopathy suggested by the presence of intraretinal microvascular abnormalities (IRMAs) and dark blot haemorrhages suggestive of retinal ischaemia.

Table 4.2 Grading system used for screening for diabetic retinopathy (UK National Guidelines)

Retinopathy (R)

Level **R0:** (no visible retinopathy)

Level **R1:** Background diabetic retinopathy (BDR) – mild

The presence of at least one of any of the following features anywhere:

- Dot haemorrhages
- Microaneurysms
- Hard exudates
- Cotton wool spots
- Blot haemorrhages
- Superficial/flame shaped haemorrhages

Level **R2:** Background diabetic retinopathy (BDR) – observable

- Four or more blot haemorrhages in one hemi-field only (inferior and superior hemi-fields delineated by a line passing through the centre of the fovea and optic disc)

Level **R3:** Background diabetic retinopathy (BDR) – referable

Any of the following features:

- Four or more blot haemorrhages in both inferior and superior hemi-fields
- Venous beading
- Intraretinal microvascular abnormalities

Level **R4:** Proliferative diabetic retinopathy (PDR) – referable

Any of the following features:

- Active new vessels
- Vitreous haemorrhage

Level **R5:** Blind or phthisical eye

Level **R6:** Not adequately visualised

- Retina not sufficiently visible for assessment – technical failure

(Continued)

Table 4.2 Grading system used for screening for diabetic retinopathy (UK National Guidelines)—Cont'd

Maculopathy (M)

Level **M0:** No maculopathy

No features ≤ 2 disc diameters (DD) from the centre of the fovea sufficient to qualify for M1 or M2 as defined below

Level **M1:** Lesions as specified below within a radius of > 1 but ≤ 2 DD from the centre of the fovea

Level **M2:** Lesions as specified below within a radius of ≤ 1 DD of the centre of the fovea

- Blot haemorrhages
- Hard exudates

Photocoagulation (P)

Laser photocoagulation scars present

Other lesions (OL)

Other non-diabetic lesions present:
- Pigmented lesion (naevus)
- Age-related macular degeneration
- Drusen maculopathy
- Myelinated nerve fibres
- Asteroid hyalosis
- Retinal vein thrombosis

Table 4.3 Guidelines for referral for specialist assessment of diabetic retinopathy

Clinical problem	Urgency
There is sudden loss of vision	Within 1 day
There is evidence of retinal detachment	Within 1 day
There is new vessel formation (on the disc or elsewhere)	Within 1 week
There is vitreous or pre-retinal haemorrhage	Within 1 week
Rubeosis iridis is present	Within 1 week
There are hard exudates within 1 DD of the fovea or clinically significant macular oedema	Within 4 weeks
There is an unexplained drop in visual acuity	Within 4 weeks
There are unexplained retinal findings	Within 4 weeks
Severe or very severe non-proliferative retinopathy is present	Within 4 weeks

General principles of management of diabetic retinopathy
Glycaemic control

Improvement of glycaemic control has been shown to reduce the risk of development and progression of diabetic retinopathy. The Diabetes Control and Complications Study (DCCT) demonstrated that intensive glycaemic control reduces the risk of onset of diabetic retinopathy, progression of pre-existing retinopathy, and the need for laser photocoagulation of patients with type 1 diabetes. The United Kingdom Prospective Diabetes Study (UKPDS) demonstrated a similar reduction in the risk of onset and progression in diabetic retinopathy in patients with type 2 diabetes.

Control of blood pressure

The UKPDS demonstrated that the risk of progression of diabetic retinopathy was decreased with tight control of blood pressure (with either captopril or atenolol) and led to an almost 35% relative reduction in the need for retinal photocoagulation. The EURODIAB Controlled Trial of Lisinopril in Insulin-dependent Diabetes (EUCLID) study (using lisinopril), and the Diabetic Retinopathy Candesartan Trials (DIRECT trial) demonstrated delay in the progression of retinopathy using drugs that act on the renin–angiotensin–aldosterone axis.

Management of dyslipidaemia

The Early Treatment Diabetic Retinopathy Study (ETDRS) and the DCCT revealed that an elevated serum cholesterol level was related to development and progression of diabetic retinopathy, especially diabetic maculopathy. Recent studies suggest that aggressive lipid lowering is beneficial in the prevention of progression and also in the management of diabetic retinopathy, especially maculopathy.

Multifactorial risk reduction

The Steno 2 trial showed benefit of multiple interventions, which included behavioural therapy (dietary intervention, exercise and smoking cessation) and pharmacological intervention (reduction of blood pressure, improvement in glycaemic control and lipid modification).

Proliferative diabetic retinopathy

Proliferative diabetic retinopathy (PDR) affects about 5–10% of the diabetic population and is more common in type 1 diabetes.

Neovascularisation is the hallmark of PDR. New vessels are commonly seen along the retinal arcades but can occur at the optic disc or elsewhere in the retina. As a general rule, the retina distal to the neovascularisation should be considered as ischaemic. It has been estimated that over one-quarter of the retina has to be non-perfused before neovascularisation occurs. Ischaemia upregulates the vascular endothelial growth factor (VEGF) in the retina, which in turn stimulates neovascularisation. New vessels start as endothelial proliferations, and pass through the internal limiting membrane to lie in the potential plane between the retina and the posterior vitreous face.

PDR can result in visual deterioration from ischaemia, haemorrhage and tractional retinal detachment involving the macula. New vessels can break through the internal limiting membrane and grow into the vitreous gel using the posterior face of the vitreous as a scaffold. This invariably leads to a pre-retinal or vitreous haemorrhage and also increases the risk of tractional retinal detachment.

Basic principles of management of diabetic retinopathy have already been discussed in previous sections. Patients with proliferative diabetic retinopathy have to be assessed and managed by specialists and are treated with panretinal photocoagulation (discussed in the following sections in detail).

New vessels ——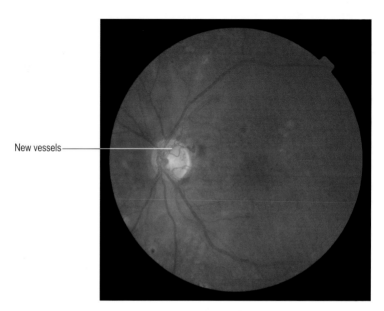

Neovascularisation at the optic disc, if present, is diagnostic of proliferative diabetic retinopathy.

Diabetic maculopathy

Involvement of the macula with exudative or ischaemic changes has a potential to involve the fovea, thus threatening vision. Exudative maculopathy may be amenable to treatment but ischaemic changes are not. Diabetic maculopathy can present in the following patterns:

- *Focal*: Focal leakage, characterised usually by the presence of a cluster of microaneurysms surrounded by retinal thickening and a complete or incomplete ring of hard exudates.

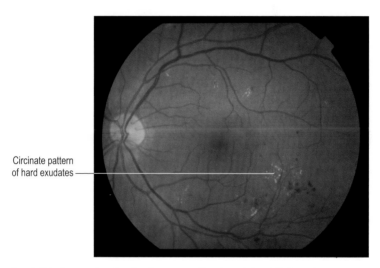

Circinate pattern of hard exudates —

Focal diabetic maculopathy showing areas of hard exudates at the macula.

- *Diffuse*: Diffuse retinal thickening and exudation from capillaries, often involving the fovea. Cystoid changes suggest chronicity of the condition.

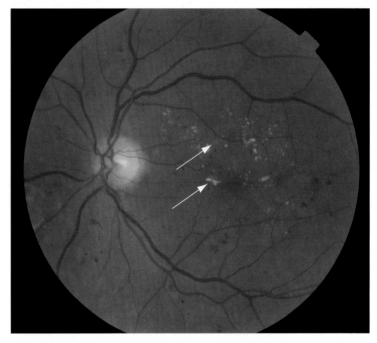

Diffuse diabetic maculopathy showing widespread hard exudates at the macula; note the paler appearance of the macula suggesting retinal thickening.

- *Ischaemic*: Diagnosed ideally by fluorescein angiography, representing an enlarged or irregular foveal avascular zone. Clinically it may lack features; however the hallmarks are reduced visual acuity, deep blot haemorrhages and IRMAs.

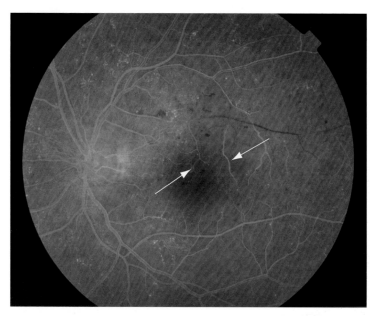

Ischaemic maculopathy. Note the disruption of the perifoveal capillary network resulting in an irregular and widened foveal avascular zone (FAZ) and adjoining areas of capillary non-perfusion.

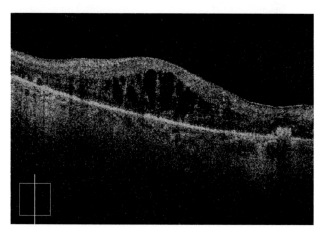

Optical coherence tomographic image showing cystoid macular oedema.

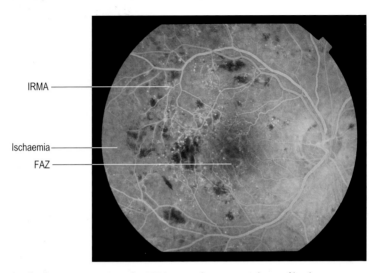

IRMA —

Ischaemia —

FAZ —

Fundus fluorescein angiographic (FFA) image showing retinal nerve fibre layer haemorrhage and deep blot haemorrhage. Temporal to the macula there are areas of capillary drop-out, intraretinal microvascular abnormalities (IRMA) representing ischaemia. The foveal avascular zone (FAZ) is enlarged and irregular, showing loss of the perifoveal capillary network.

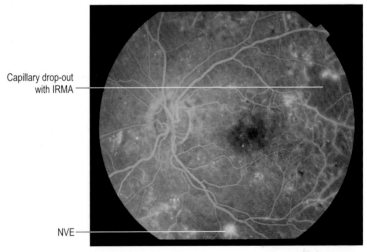

Capillary drop-out
with IRMA —

NVE —

FFA image showing proliferative changes such as neovascularisation elsewhere (NVE) in the retina. Intraretinal microvascular abnormalities (IRMA).

Laser photocoagulation

The efficacy of photocoagulation has been demonstrated in the ETDRS study. It is believed that the regression of neovascularisation is due to the destruction of the ischaemic and hypoxic retina with the reduction in angiogenic factors.

Panretinal photocoagulation is now the main modality of treatment for proliferative diabetic retinopathy and severe non-proliferative diabetic retinopathy. Clinically significant macular oedema (CSMO) can be treated with focal or grid photocoagulation.

Panretinal laser involves the application of 500 μm of Argon laser photocoagulation spots, each separated by an interval of a similar spot size to the mid-peripheral retina. A row of laser burns is initially placed approximately three disc diameters temporal to the fovea to avoid getting too close to the fovea. About 1500 burns are usually required (in two or three sessions). Severe cases may require further photocoagulation. The aim is to cover the ischaemic areas, and regression of new vessels occurs in almost 80% of cases. Fundus fluorescein angiography (FFA) could be done initially to delineate the ischaemic areas; however, it should be done to ensure coverage of ischaemic areas with the laser if good regression of neovascularisation is not achieved with initial retinal photocoagulation.

Laser treatment can be associated with pain, transient visual loss, loss of visual field (inevitable) and sometimes reduced visual acuity and choroidal damage.

In very aggressive cases of PDR, an intravitreal injection of an anti-VEGF can give a valuable window period while waiting for laser photocoagulation to take effect which can take up to 2 weeks.

Examples of newer and older types of laser treatment

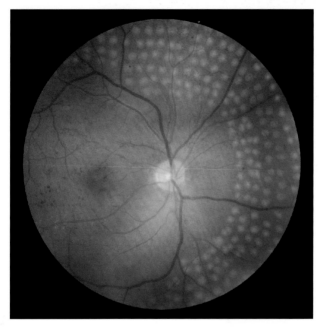

Fresh laser burns applied as part of panretinal photocoagulation.

Fresh laser burns appear greyish white. Laser energy is taken up by the pigment in the retinal pigment epithelium, resulting in photocoagulation or a thermal burn of the retina. Within a period of about 2 weeks the laser burns appear hyperpigmented. The above image shows fresh laser burns applied as part of a panretinal photocoagulation.

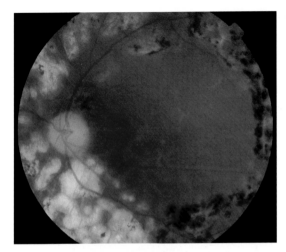

Older laser burns (larger spot size) appear more intense due to the larger and stronger thermal reaction caused by the application.

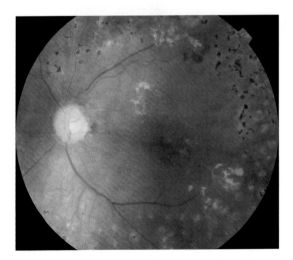

Regression of neovascularisation following panretinal photocoagulation. Note the much smaller spot sizes of newer laser burns.

Macular laser

Laser photocoagulation is considered primarily for clinically significant macular oedema. This could be applied focally to leaking microaneurysms or in a grid pattern over the macula in cases of diffuse macular oedema. The spot sizes used vary from 50 to 100 μ and power just enough to cause a very minimal blanch. Using higher power by itself can result in reduction of visual acuity. Utmost care should be taken to avoid the foveal avascular zone (FAZ). Ideally a macular laser should be done only after angiographically assessing the macula.

Other modalities in the local management of macular oedema are intravitreal injections of triamcinolone acetonide or anti-VEGF. However, the effect of these is only short-lived.

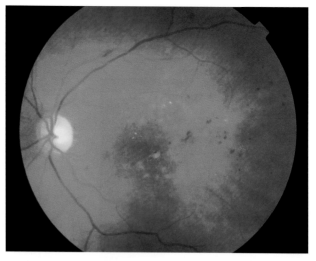

Grid laser burns are applied in a grid fashion to the macula, avoiding the foveal avascular zone.

Grid laser burns are applied in a grid fashion to the macula, avoiding the FAZ. These mild laser burns help to stimulate the retinal pigment epithelium to dry the macular oedema by actively pumping the fluid out of the retina.

Focal laser burns are targeted at the leaky microaneurysm within a circinate area of hard exudate.

CHAPTER 5

Hypertensive Retinopathy

The primary response of retinal arterioles to systemic hypertension is narrowing. The degree of narrowing is dependent upon the amount of pre-existing arteriosclerosis (see Box 5.1). For this reason hypertensive narrowing is seen in its pure form only in young individuals.

Hypertensive retinopathy is characterised by:

- *Vasoconstriction*, which can be generalised or focal with arteriolar narrowing. However, ophthalmoscopic diagnosis of generalised narrowing may be difficult.
- *Leakage*, which is caused by abnormal vascular permeability leading to the development of flame-shaped haemorrhages, hard exudates and a retinal oedema. Swelling of the optic nerve is the hallmark of malignant phase hypertension.
- *Arteriosclerosis*, which is caused by thickening of the vessel wall, which consists of intimal hyalinization and medial hypertrophy. With increased thickening of arterial wall and narrowing of lumen, the light diffuses giving rise to a 'copper wire' reflex. When this process continues it assumes a 'silver wire' appearance when the blood is no longer visualised. Arteriosclerosis also leads to changes at the arteriovenous crossing termed as 'AV nipping'. This can vary from tapering of vein (venous compression 'Gunn's sign' on either side of the crossing to interruption of visible column of blood.

Box 5.1 Keith–Wagener–Barker classification of hypertensive retinopathy

Grade 1

Mild to moderate narrowing or sclerosis of the arteries

Grade 2

Moderate to marked narrowing of the arterioles
Local and/or generalised narrowing of arterioles
Exaggeration of the light reflex
Arteriovenous crossing changes

Grade 3

Retinal arteriolar narrowing and focal constriction
Retinal oedema
Cotton wool patches
Haemorrhage

Grade 4

As for Grade 3, plus papilloedema

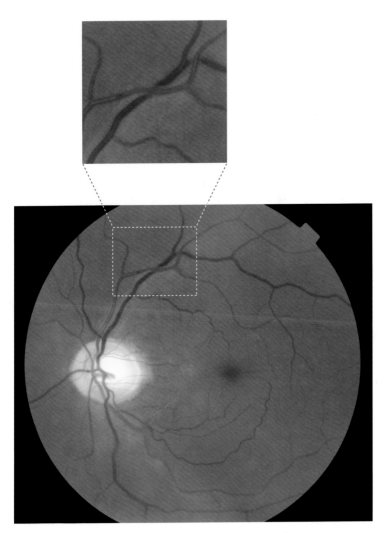

Arteriovenous nipping secondary to hypertensive retinopathy. At the arteriovenous crossing the vessels share a common sheath within which the hardened artery, secondary to arteriosclerotic changes, compresses the retinal vein.

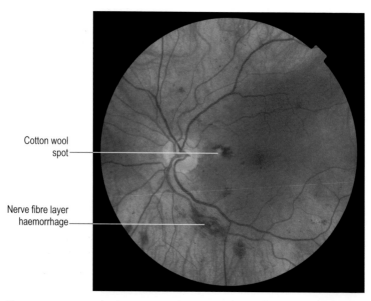

Cotton wool spot ———

Nerve fibre layer haemorrhage ———

Hypertensive retinopathy showing nerve fibre layer (pre-retinal) haemorrhage and cotton wool spot secondary to interruption of axoplasmic flow representing nerve fibre layer infarcts.

Management of hypertension

Non-pharmacological treatment of high blood pressure

The following lifestyle measures should be recommended for all patients with high blood pressure:

- Reduce salt intake.
- Limit alcohol consumption: less than 21 units/week for men and 14 units/week for women is recommended.
- Lose weight: people with hypertension who are overweight (body mass index [BMI] 25–30) or obese (BMI > 30) should be encouraged to lose weight.
- Increase physical exercise.
- Follow a healthy diet: a randomized trial found that patients who increased fruit and vegetable consumption to at least five portions a day showed a significant reduction in blood pressure of approximately 4/1.5 mmHg. Other healthy eating suggestions include replacing saturated fat with polyunsaturated and monounsaturated fats, eating oily fish and reducing total fat intake.
- Stop smoking.

Pharmacological treatment of high blood pressure

If the lifestyle measures outlined above are ineffective in reducing a patient's high blood pressure to acceptable levels, the British Hypertension Society recommends a four-step treatment programme as outlined in the following algorithm.

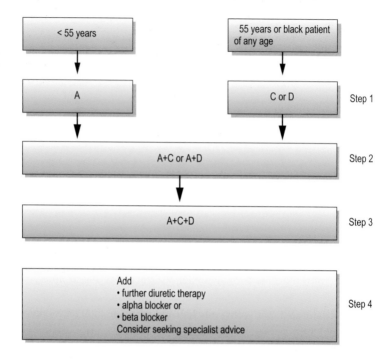

A = ACE inhibitor
C = Calcium channel blocker
D = Diuretic

The British Hypertension Society (BHS) A/CD algorithm for the treatment of high blood pressure. A, angiotensin converting enzyme inhibitor; C, calcium channel blocker; D, diuretic. Redrawn from BHS IV Summary. BMJ 2004; 328: 634–640.

Papilloedema

Papilloedema is defined as the swelling of the optic nerve head secondary to raised intracranial pressure. It is bilateral, although it may be asymmetrical. As the term 'papilloedema' is reserved for raised intracranial pressure all other causes of a swollen optic disc are referred to as disc swelling.

Patients with papilloedema should be suspected of having an intracranial mass until proved to the contrary. However, if anatomical variation at the optic nerve exists, papilloedema may not develop even if the intracranial pressure is raised. Since chronic papilloedema results in glial scarring of the optic nerve head, patients who have had a subsequent rise in intracranial pressure need not develop fresh papilloedema.

Causes of raised intracranial pressure

- Space-occupying lesion.
- Blockage of the ventricular system (by congenital or acquired lesions).
- Obstruction of cerebrospinal fluid (CSF) absorption (via arachnoid villi, previously damaged by meningitis).

- Subarachnoid haemorrhage or cerebral trauma.
- Idiopathic intracranial hypertension.
- Diffuse cerebral oedema (possibly from blunt head trauma).
- Severe hypertension.
- Very rarely by hypersecretion of CSF by a choroidal plexus tumour.

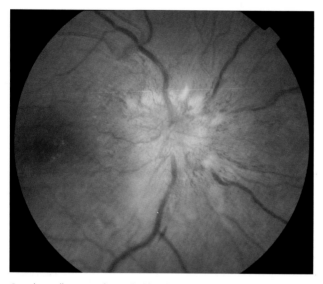

Grossly swollen optic disc with dilated vessels and flame haemorrhage. The normal cup is totally obliterated and cotton wool spots are present at the peripapillary region due to interruption of axoplasmic flow in the retinal nerve axons. Although there may be transient loss of vision, permanent visual deterioration only occurs late with an enlarged blind spot.

CHAPTER 7

Optic Atrophy

Optic atrophy is a hallmark of damage to the retinal ganglion cells. Clinically it is seen as pallor of the optic disc. This change usually takes weeks to develop after the insult has occurred. It is associated with loss of vision.

Classically, optic atrophy has been classified as primary, secondary and consecutive:

- In primary optic atrophy pallor occurs without prior optic disc swelling and is seen as a consequence of retrobulbar damage to the optic nerve up to the lateral geniculate body. The optic disc appears whiter than usual with well-defined margins.
- In secondary optic atrophy, optic disc swelling is seen prior to pallor. The optic disc margins may appear less defined and the colour appears dirty white to grey.
- Consecutive optic atrophy is a consequence of diffuse retinal disease and, in addition to the findings as described in secondary optic atrophy, the retina appears abnormal.

Aetiology

- Hereditary autosomal dominant or autosomal recessive optic atrophy.
- Leber heriditary optic neuropathy.
- Retinal dystrophy including retinitis pigmentosa.

- Vascular causes include central retinal artery occlusion which is often associated with other evidence of vascular disease.
- Nutritional causes include vitamin B_{12} deficiency.
- Other causes include tobacco, alcohol and drugs (e.g. ethambutol).
- Inflammatory causes include sarcoidosis and polyarteritis nodosa.
- In patients with demyelination there is often a history of attacks of optic neuritis and other neurological symptoms.
- Compressive causes include optic nerve glioma, meningioma or other intracranial tumours.

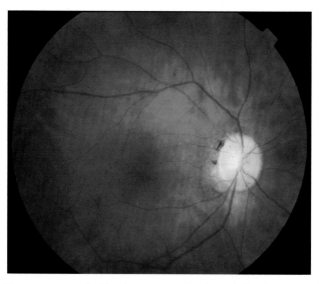

Primary optic atrophy. The disc appears pale, almost chalky white, with well-defined margins.

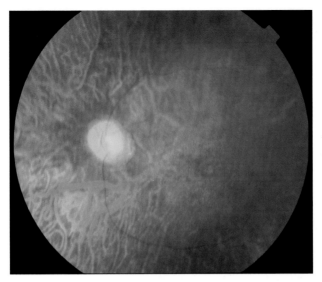

Secondary optic atrophy. Note the dirty white appearance of the optic disc with poorly defined margins, thready retinal vessels and diffuse retinal atrophy.

CHAPTER 8

Glaucoma

Glaucoma is a disease which results in progressive optic neuropathy due to a variety of risk factors. It is classified into open angle, angle closure and glaucoma due to developmental anomalies. It can be further divided into primary open or primary angle closure glaucoma or secondary causes resulting in either.

Three features that are the hallmark of glaucoma are:

1. Raised intraocular pressure (normal range 10–21 mmHg),
2. Progressive optic neuropathy represented by an enlargement of the optic cup, and
3. A corresponding progressive visual field defect as a consequence of the above.

If untreated, glaucoma results in irreversible blindness.

The only proven effective treatment is reduction of intraocular pressure, initially medically and later, if required, surgically. The definitive treatment for acute primary angle closure glaucoma following medical reduction of intraocular pressure is to create a hole in the peripheral iris (iridotomy) usually by laser, which prevents an angle closure in the future.

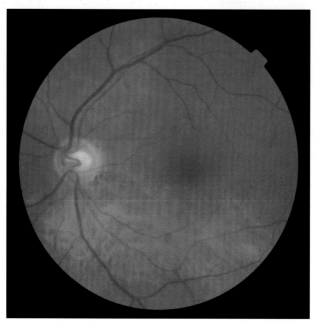

Glaucoma. Note enlargement of the optic cup due to thinning of the neuroretinal rim caused by loss of retinal nerve fibres.

CHAPTER 9

Retinal Vascular Occlusions

Retinal artery occlusion

Embolisation is a common cause for retinal arterial obstruction however it may also be caused by inflammation. The task of the clinician is to find the cause and in the case of emboli, the source.

Heart

Emboli from the heart may be from:

- Thrombus originating from the left side of the heart as a consequence of a mural thrombus secondary to myocardial infarction or atrial fibrillation.
- Calcific emboli from the mitral or aortic valve
- Vegetations from valves due to bacterial endocarditis
- Cardiac myxoma in rare cases

Internal carotid artery

The bifurcation of the common carotid artery into the external and internal carotid arteries is vulnerable to atherosclerosis. Emboli from the carotid artery or the heart may be of the following types:

- *Cholesterol emboli* appear as minute refractile gold into yellow crystals. They often appear at arteriolar bifurcations and as they rarely cause significant obstruction are generally asymptomatic.

- *Fibrin-platelet emboli* are dull and plaque like in appearance. They may be the cause of retinal transient ischaemic attack (TIA – amaurosis fugax) and occasionally complete obstruction. The patient will complain of painless unilateral loss of vision, often described as a curtain coming down. The visual loss usually lasts for a few minutes and spontaneous recovery follows. Frequency may range from several times a day to one every few months.
- *Calcific emboli* appear as a larger, white, non-refractile, usually single embolus near the optic nerve. They may cause complete obstruction of the artery resulting in loss of vision.

Other causes of embolus are from intravenous drug abuse or lipid embolus due to pancreatitis.

Inflammatory diseases such as Systemic lupus erythematosus, Polyarteritis nodosa, Wagener's granulomatosis, Behcet's disease and Giant cell arteritis can cause retinal arterial obstruction.

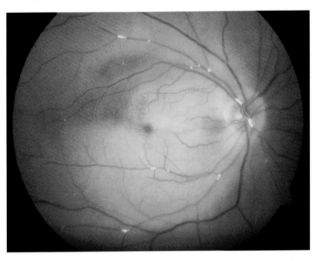

Central retinal artery occlusion. Note the multiple retinal artery emboli and ischaemic retina suggested by diffuse pallor of the posterior pole.

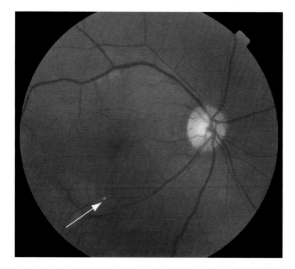

Branch retinal artery occlusion. Note the occluding plaque in the inferotemporal retinal artery. The artery beyond appears narrowed with a broken column of blood. The affected retina appears pale, suggesting ischaemia, whereas the normal colour of the fundus is preserved in the unaffected retina.

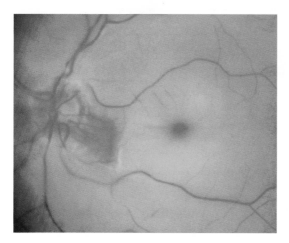

Central retinal artery occlusion with cherry red spot. Note the diffuse retinal ischaemia represented by the pale retina. The fovea retains its normal red reflex (cherry red spot) since it has only photoreceptors and is devoid of any overlying inner retinal layers.

Retinal venous occlusion

The retinal artery and vein share a common sheath at the optic nerve head and at the site of arteriovenous crossing. The retinal artery which hardens with age tends to compress the vein beside it at the optic nerve head or at the crossing sites especially if the arteriole crosses over the vein. Narrowing of the vein eventually leads to the formation of a thrombus and occlusion. This results in raised capillary pressure and rupture causing haemorrhages and retinal oedema. Stagnation of blood results in secondary retinal ischaemia.

Central retinal vein occlusion

This presents clinically as an acute unilateral impairment of vision, the profoundness depending on the amount of ischaemia.

Features seen are:
- Extensive nerve fibre layer and dot and blot haemorrhages
- Tortuous, enlarged retinal veins
- Optic disc swelling
- Cotton wool spots
- Macular oedema.

Risk factors – including hypertension, diabetes mellitus, hyperviscosity and glaucoma – must be identified and treated if present. If the retina becomes ischaemic it stimulates the formation of new vessels on the iris (rubeosis) and subsequent neovascularisation of the angle may lead to secondary glaucoma. Fluorescein angiography may be useful. Laser treatment may be used to ablate the ischaemic retina in an attempt to prevent new vessel formation.

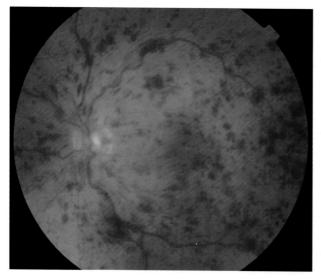

Central retinal vein occlusion. Note the scattered, flame-shaped, nerve fibre layer and deeper blot haemorrhages all over the retina with tortuous, dilated retinal veins. The normal appearance of the macula is lost due to oedema.

Branch retinal vein occlusion

Significant visual loss usually accompanies occlusion of temporal retinal veins which also drain the macula. Haemorrhage occurs along the area of retina drained by the occluded vein.

Chronic signs include cystoid macular oedema which may be accompanied by underlying retinal pigment epithelial atrophy. Veins show sheathing and arterioles are often narrowed.

Visual recovery depends on the formation of collateral vessels which re-route the drainage of blood to normalise capillary pressure.

Poor vision results due to chronic macular oedema, macular ischaemia and neovascularisation secondary to ischaemia.

Prompt laser photocoagulation to the ischaemic retina is required to prevent vitreous haemorrhage and neovascular glaucoma.

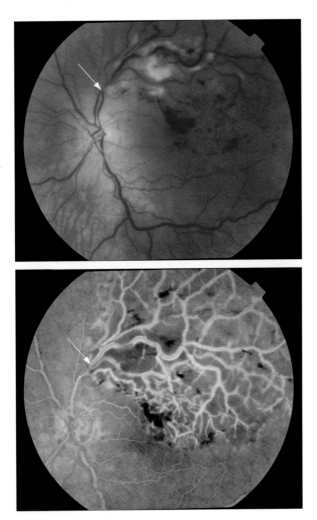

Branch retinal vein occlusion. The colour image shows a dilated tortuous superotemporal vein with cotton wool spots and haemorrhages in the affected retina. Note the site of occlusion is where the artery crosses over the retinal vein (arrowhead). The fluorescein angiographic image shows the darker ischaemic retina. The haemorrhage at the macula masks the fluorescence.

CHAPTER 10

Fundal Haemorrhages

Vitreous haemorrhage

Haemorrhage into the vitreous can result in painless loss of vision. The extent of the visual loss will depend on the degree of haemorrhage. Small haemorrhages may be asymptomatic or present with floaters and/or a slight reduction in visual acuity.

Haemorrhage may be due to traction on the fragile new vessels, usually due to proliferative diabetic retinopathy, a retinal tear avulsing a retinal blood vessel, traumatic or breakthrough of a subretinal haemorrhage into the vitreous.

Urgent referral to an ophthalmologist is important to determine the cause and manage any complications.

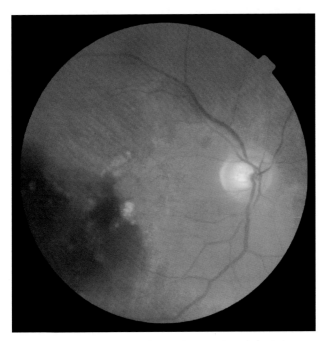

Vitreous haemorrhage. Note the haemorrhage masking the underlying retinal vessels.

Subhyaloid haemorrhage

This haemorrhage settles behind the posterior face of the vitreous gel but in front of the retina. It usually takes a boat shape with a flat superior border and a crescent-shaped inferior border. It occludes the retinal details as it lies in front of it. It usually arises from neovascularisation secondary to proliferative diabetic retinopathy but may also result from trauma or rupture of a retinal artery macroaneurysm. It usually takes much longer to absorb than an intragel vitreous haemorrhage and may require surgical clearance if it lies in front of the macula.

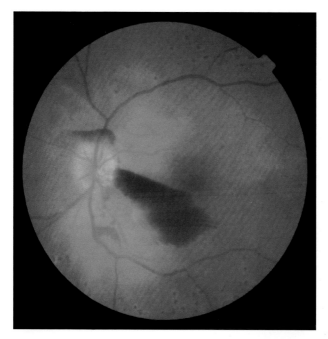

Subhyaloid haemorrhage. Note the haemorrhage masking the underlying features. It usually takes a boat shape with a straight superior border and a curved inferior border. Note neovascularisation at optic disc.

CHAPTER 11

Age-Related Macular Degeneration

Age-related macular degeneration (ARMD) is the result of a spectrum of changes that occur at the macula seen in individuals over the age of 50 years. The incidence increases from 3.9% in those aged 43–54 years to 22.8% in those aged 75 years and over (Beaver Dam Eye Study).

Drusen

Early changes are seen as deposits under the retinal pigment epithelium (RPE) called drusen. These appear as yellow excrescences in the posterior pole. They may vary in number, size, shape, degree of elevation and extent of associated changes in the RPE. Drusen are rarely clinically visible before the age of 45 years but are fairly common between the ages of 45 and 60 years and almost always thereafter.

Types of ARMD

There are two main types of ARMD: non-exudative and exudative.

Non-exudative ARMD

Non-exudative ARMD is slowly progressive with mild to moderate impairment of central vision developing over several months or years. It accounts for 90% of cases.

It usually presents with focal hyperpigmentation of the RPE followed by development of the sharply circumscribed circular areas of RPE atrophy (geographic atrophy) associated with varying degrees of loss of choriocapillaris. Subsequently, the larger choroidal vessels may become prominent within the atrophic areas and pre-existing drusen may disappear.

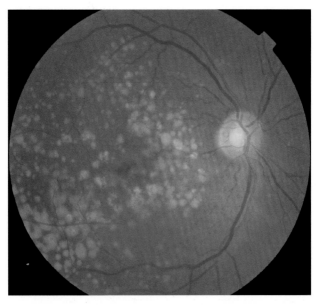

Hallmarks of dry ARMD. Small hard and larger soft and confluent drusen are seen at the macula along with hyperpigmentation of RPE.

One or both eyes may be affected; when bilateral, the lesions are frequently symmetrical. Unfortunately, treatment is not available although the provision of low vision aids is useful in many patients. AREDS (Age Related Eye Disease Study) is looking into effects of supplementing Leutein 10mg, Zeaxanthin 2mg and Omega 3 fatty acids on the risk of progression of ARMD. Risk factors such as smoking and exposure to ultraviolet light should be addressed.

Exudative ARMD

Exudative ARMD is much less common and is rapidly progressive. In some cases vision may be lost within a few days. It may occur in isolation or in association with dry ARMD. Features of exudative ARMD are detachment of RPE and those secondary to choroidal neovascularisation such as sub-retinal haemorrhage, sub retinal fluid and hard exudates. Treatment with intravitreal injections of anti vascular endothelial growth factors (Ranibizumab) is advised to stop progression.

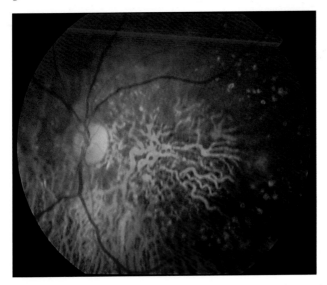

Advanced non-exudative ARMD showing geographic atrophy at the macula with larger choroidal vessels showing through. Note the surrounding calcified drusen.

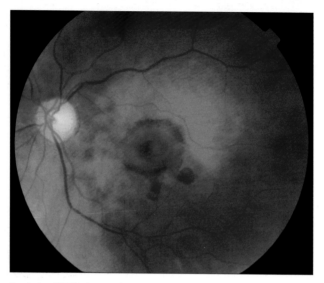

Exudative ARMD showing hyperpigmentation representing a choroidal neovascular membrane surrounded by subretinal haemorrhage.

CHAPTER 12

Lipaemia Retinalis

Lipaemia retinalis is a rare disorder characterized by the creamy white appearance of retinal blood vessels and occurs in patients with severe hypertriglyceridaemia. High levels of circulating chylomicrons account for the appearance. Normally this is not associated with visual loss and the appearance disappears when serum triglyceride returns to normal level.

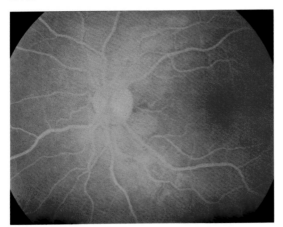

Lipaemia retinalis. Note the creamy white appearance of the retinal blood vessels due to hypertriglyceridaemia.

CHAPTER 13

Angioid Streaks

Angioid streaks appear as dark red or brown irregular lines radiating from the optic disc. They represent cracks or dehiscence in Bruch's membrane which is thickened and calcified. There is a risk of secondary choroidal neovascularisation developing through these cracks, which can result in visual loss if it involves the fovea. Neovascularisation can be treated with anti-vascular endothelial growth factor (anti-VEGF) agents although the risks of scarring and recurrence are high.

The systemic disease with which this is most commonly associated is pseudoxanthoma elasticum. An associated fundus finding of peau d'orange is seen as a fine stippled appearance at the interface of the lighter orange colour at the area of the crack with the darker orange colour of the normal fundus.

Other systemic conditions associated with angioid streaks are Paget's disease, sickle cell anaemia and Ehlers–Danlos syndrome. Ehlers–Danlos syndrome is a rare, usually dominantly inherited, disorder of collagen. Systemic features include thin skin which is hyperelastic and heals poorly. Joints are hyperextensible. Bleeding diatheses and dissecting aneurysms may occur. Other lesions include diaphragmatic hernias, diverticula of the upper gastrointestinal and respiratory tracts, as well as epicanthic folds, high myopia and retinal detachment.

Angioid streaks

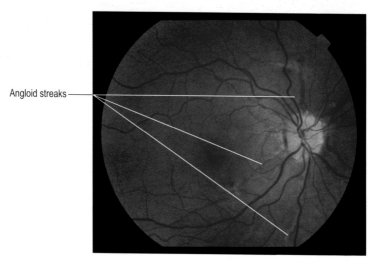

Angioid streaks. Note the radiating dark, irregular streaks from the optic disc.

CHAPTER 14

Retinitis Pigmentosa

Retinitis pigmentosa is a term used for a group of hereditary disorders that are characterised by a progressive loss of photoreceptor and retinal pigment epithelium function. The prevalence is approximately 1:5000.

Inheritance

- Approximately 23% are sporadic without any family history.
- Approximately 45% are autosomal dominant and have the best prognosis.
- Approximately 20% are autosomal recessive. X-linked recessive is uncommon and has the worst prognosis.
- In 6% of cases there is an uncertain family history.

Clinical signs

Retinitis pigmentosa is associated with bilateral loss of peripheral vision, caused by predominantly rod dysfunction, followed by progressive loss of cone photoreceptor function. Presentation is usually with defective dark adaptation (night blindness). By the third decade over

75% of patients are symptomatic. The age of onset, clinical progression, visual loss and the presence of clinical features are usually related to the form of inheritance.

Progressive constriction of the peripheral visual field ultimately leads to tunnel vision which may eventually be lost. Classic clinical features are represented by arteriolar narrowing, perivascular bone spicule pigmentation and a waxy optic disc pallor. Advanced feature suggesting atrophy may present as unmasking of larger choroidal vessels.

Other associations commonly are cataract, open-angle glaucoma, cystoid macular oedema, keratoconus and myopia. Systemic associations are Refsum syndrome, Barder-Biedl syndrome, Kearns-Sayre syndrome and Bassen-Kornzweig syndrome.

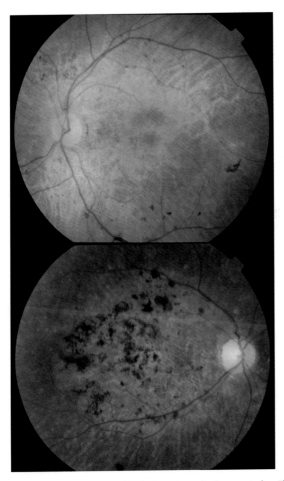

Retinitis pigmentosa. Note the dark, perivascular bone spicules. The optic disc appears pale with thready retinal blood vessels. The upper image shows loss of the foveal reflex at the macula; the lower image shows advanced changes with hyperpigmentation, macular atrophy and unmasking of larger choroidal vessels.

CHAPTER 15

Choroidal Naevus

Choroidal naevi are benign single or occasionally multiple grey or bluish lesions. They are round or oval and are usually less than 5 mm in diameter. They are usually present at birth and tend to grow until the end of puberty. If there is any increase in size or pigmentation in adulthood, then the possibility of malignant change should be considered. The benign lesions are asymptomatic, except rarely when a macular lesion can lead to a serous retinal detachment (see overleaf). Presence of drusen is a favourable sign to stay benign whereas haemorrhage, fluid or lipofuscin are not.

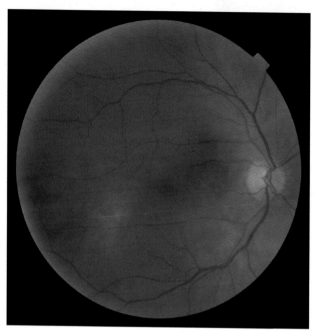

Choroidal naevus. Note the bluish-grey area of discoloration with indistinct margins. The overlying retina appears normal.

Melanocytoma

Melanocytomas may arise anywhere in the uveal tract. In the anterior segment acute necrosis of the tumour may cause inflammation, pigment dispersion and secondary glaucoma. Most frequently melanocytomas affect the optic nerve head. They typically affect dark-skinned individuals but may also occur in whites. Detection is usually by chance, although occasionally a deep-seated tumour causes optic nerve dysfunction as a result of necrosis.

Clinical signs

Melanocytoma presents as a black lesion with feathery edges, most frequently occupying the inferior part of the optic nerve head. Occasionally the tumour is elevated and occupies the entire disc surface, and a small proportion develop into melanomas. It is uncertain whether these represent melanomas in the first place or whether they are initially melanocytomas that undergo malignant transformation.

Treatment

Treatment is not required except in the very rare event of malignant transformation.

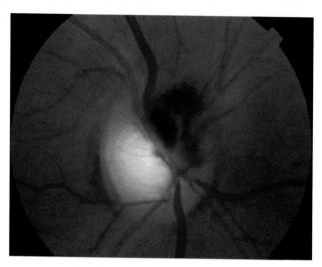

Melanocytoma. Note the dark raised lesion bordering the superonasal part of the optic disc with feathery margins.

CHAPTER 17

Ocular Inflammation

Choroiditis/chorioretinitis

Although the term choroiditis signifies inflammation of the choroid, it often involves the overlying retina resulting in chorioretinitis. The causes are either infectious or inflammatory.

Infectious causes

- Toxoplasmosis
- Toxocariasis
- Tuberculosis
- Syphilis
- Ocular histoplasmosis

Inflammatory causes

- Sarcoidosis
- Birdshot choroidopathy
- Punctate inner choroidopathy
- Sympathetic ophthalmia

Clinical signs

Clinically the lesions may be single or multiple, varying from 1 disc diameter to less in size. Inactive lesions appear as well-delineated, hypopigmented patches with hyperpigmented clumps and borders.

Active lesions appear poorly delineated, with fuzzy margins and overlying inflammation; oedema gives a pale white cloudy appearance. In toxoplasmosis an active lesion is usually seen adjacent to an old inactive one. Inflammatory cells may also be seen in the vitreous, making the media hazy. If a lesion affects the fovea, it can result in significant loss of central vision.

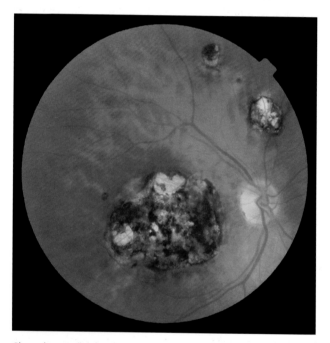

Choroiditis. Well-defined inactive lesions with clear areas showing the sclera interspersed with dark areas of choroidal pigment.

Cytomegalovirus retinitis

Cytomegalovirus resides in the body, usually as a commensal. However, in an immunocompromised state (AIDS, severe immunosuppression in inflammatory disease, aplastic anaemia) it can result in infections of the retina.

Clinical signs

Retinitis is seen typically along the blood vessels and looks like white cottage cheese (representing a necrotic retina) with ketchup (retinal haemorrhage). It may be seen at the optic disc or in the peripheral retina. The vitreous is usually clear due to the individual being unable to

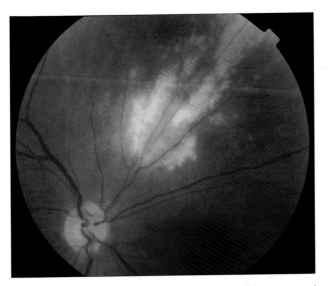

Cytomegalovirus retinitis. Cottage cheese appearance of the superonasal perivascular retina representing areas of active retinitis. These areas later become atrophic. At this stage they are prone to developing retinal tears.

host an immunological response. It can spread rapidly and can result in loss of vision due to involvement of the fovea, vascular occlusion or secondary retinal detachment.

Treatment

Treatment is in the form of either systemic administration or intravitreal injection of ganciclovir.

CHAPTER 18

Roth Spot

Roth spots are retinal haemorrhages with a pale white centre and rarely involve the macula. Histologically, they consist of platelet and fibrin thrombus in the centre surrounded by haemorrhage from a ruptured retinal capillary.

Although initially described in subacute bacterial endocarditis, they are non-specific and can occur in other conditions such as blood dyscrasias, diabetic and hypertensive retinopathy, severe anaemia, shaken baby syndrome and anoxia. They are asymptomatic and usually resolve when the cause is treated.

Roth spot ———

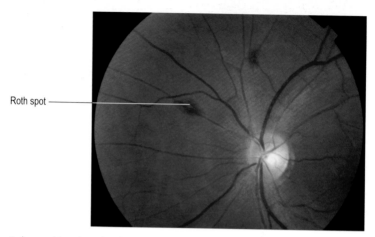

Roth spot. Note the pale white centre of this lesion nasal to the optic disc.

CHAPTER 19

Retinal Detachment

Separation of the neurosensory retina from the retinal pigment epithelium is termed retinal detachment (RD). It is classified into three types: rhegmatogenous, exudative and tractional.

Rhegmatogenous retinal detachment

Rhegmatogenous RD is caused by a retinal tear that allows the vitreous gel to access the subretinal space and detach the retina. Presenting symptoms are floaters, flashes and visual field defect.

If very small and isolated, argon laser retinopexy could be done to create a scar around the tear to prevent further progression.

Choices of surgery are either in the form of an external procedure of cryotherapy to the tear to create a scar and scleral buckle to indent the globe so as to close the tear and prevent further traction from the vitreous gel, or an intraocular procedure with vitrectomy and laser around the retinal tear.

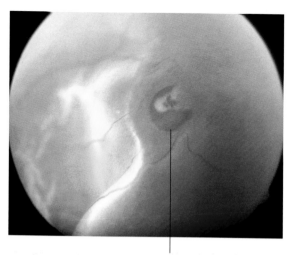

Horseshoe retinal tear

Rhegmatogenous retinal detachment. Note the horseshoe retinal tear with surrounding detached retina. The detached retina appears grey and thrown into folds.

Exudative retinal detachment

Exudative RD is due to the accumulation of serous fluid in the sub-retinal space without a retinal tear. The retinal pigment epithelial cell pump is damaged, usually due to inflammation (Harada disease, posterior scleritis). Management is by treating the cause.

Tractional retinal detachment

Tractional RD is due to pre-retinal tractional bands pulling the neurosensory retina away from the retinal pigment epithelium. The most common cause is fibrovascular proliferation due to proliferative diabetic retinopathy or trauma. If the detachment involves the macula, it can result in loss of vision.

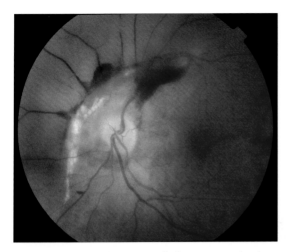

Traumatic retinal detachment. Note the large tear nasal to the optic disc involving the retina and choroid. There are pre-retinal and subretinal haemorrhages. The peripheral nasal retina is detached, represented by the bluish area.

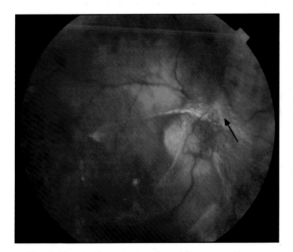

Tractional retinal detachment. Note the fibrovascular complex elevating the retina around the optic disc.

INDEX

Note: Page numbers followed by *f* indicate figures; *t* indicate tables; *b* indicate boxes.

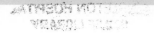